MEDICARE
BREAKDOWN
THE ALPHABET SOUP OF MEDICARE

D1522041

ISBN: 9798733532264

TABLE OF CONTENTS

PART 1
MEDICARE BREAKDOWN

$$A + B + G + D$$

$$A+B < C + HIP$$

The above two formulas probably do not mean a whole lot to someone starting down the Medicare road, but we are about to simplify the heck out of this!

I was in the Marine Corps, and the drill instructors in boot camp would call us window lickers and say they were going to break down a topic Barney style (You know, the big purple dinosaur that taught kids all sorts of stuff). Well, I am not going to call you a window licker, but I will break this down *BARNEY STYLE!*

Medicare in its current state was created by a combination of two types of people:

Economists who would never use it and *Actuarial Mathematicians* who would never have to pay for it. This dynamic duo handed us a shiny turd to deal with, but by the end of this, you'll find that Medicare isn't that bad for the Medicare beneficiary if they choose the right system from the get-go! It's that choosing that's so hard with all of the misinformation and confusing terminology.

Without further delay, I will jump right into the Alphabet Soup of Medicare and start with several things you need to understand before continuing!

THE PARTS OF MEDICARE

Medicare Has 4 Parts

Everyone goes over these, but again, I am not everyone. So, I'll tell you what you need to know!

- **PART A** — Hospital (Mostly Room and Board)

- **PART B** — Medical (Surgery, Doctors Visits, Durable Medical Equipment) Think almost all Medical treatments, procedures, labs, etc... except for hospital room and board and prescriptions.

- **PART C** — Medicare Advantage (If you choose this route you pretty much can forget about what Parts A and B cover because you no longer have them while on Part C) Think Privatized Medicare that you normally have to keep for an entire calendar year at a time. By the way, this isn't necessarily bad. It just depends on someone's particular circumstances.

- **PART D** — (Prescription Drug Plans) This one is simple. It is a standalone plan you purchase with Parts A and B or sometimes with certain Part C plans. This plan covers your drugs.

PART A

WHAT DOES MEDICARE PART A COVER?

INPATIENT HOSPITAL CARE: This includes all care you receive after being admitted into a hospital by a physician. Medicare covers up to 90 days each benefit period in a general hospital. In addition, you receive 60 lifetime reserve days. It also covers up to 190 lifetime days in a Medicare-certified psychiatric hospital.

SKILLED NURSING FACILITY CARE: Medicare covers your room, board, and certain services provided in a skilled nursing facility. This includes medications, tube feedings, and wound care. It covers up to 100 days each benefit period. To qualify, you must have spent at least three consecutive days in the hospital within 30 days of admission to a skilled nursing facility and must have needed skilled nursing or therapy services.

HOME HEALTH CARE: Though it is normally covered by Part B, Part A coverage will kick in if you have spent at least three consecutive days as a hospital inpatient within 14 days of receiving home care. Up to 100 days of daily care are covered or an unlimited amount of intermittent care.

HOSPICE CARE: Hospice care is covered for as long as your provider certifies it is necessary.

HOW MUCH DOES IT COST?

Most of the time, Part A has no cost. Certain taxes you paid during your working years are specifically for future Medicare coverage.

As long as you worked for at least 10 years in your lifetime in the United States, most of the time you won't pay a dime. If you have not, you can still purchase Part A if you've been a legal resident or have had a green card for at least five years.

Speak with one of our Medicare specialists for the latest premium costs.

HOLES IN PART A

- Part A has a hospital admission deductible that at the time of writing this (2024) is $1,632.

- Part A also has daily hospital copays that start at days 61-90 at $408 a day and on days 91-150, they go up to $816.

- Part A also has a daily copay for Skilled Nursing Care that starts on day 21 and goes through day 100. This daily copay is currently $204 per day.

PART B

Part B is much more simple. Now you recall that it covers all of the medical stuff filling in the gap on services between hospital room and board and Prescriptions.

Part B has a calendar year deductible that in 2024 is $240 ONE TIME for the calendar year. This is the amount you pay 100% of before Part B starts picking up anything.

After that deductible is met, Part B turns into 80/20 coverage. This means Part B will cover 80% of the services and you'll be responsible for 20% of the Medicare Allowable Charge. The biggest problem here is that the 20% has NO CAP.

When you're on a group plan or an ACA plan you have similar coinsurance structures, but those plans have MOOPs or Maximum out of Pockets that create a stop loss. With Parts A and B of Medicare, there is no structured stop loss.

PART C

We will break down Part C a little later on!

PART D

Part D is your prescription drug coverage, but it can be one of the most confusing or cost-prohibitive parts of coverage for Medicare beneficiaries.

There are four phases of coverage within Part D: Deductible, Initial Coverage Level, Coverage Gap AKA The Donut Hole, and the Catastrophic Phase!

The deductible for 2024 on Part D is capped at $545 although there are some plans with a $0 deductible. Typically the deductible is one of the least important aspects of a Part D equation as it normally isn't applied to Tier 1 and 2 Medications and if someone has extremely expensive medication the plans with $0 deductible normally cost $500-$600 more in annual premium, offsetting the deductible savings.

THE INITIAL COVERAGE LEVEL—It would have been too simple for Congress to have just left everyone in this level of coverage. This is where 81% of people stay throughout the year. It's based on where your drugs fall in the formulary and the corresponding copay that tier requires. Sometimes Tiers 1 and 2 are as low as $0 copay in this phase while Tiers 3, 4, and 5 warrant a higher copay and sometimes a percentage of the MSRP cost of the drug.

THE DONUT HOLE — 19% of Part D beneficiaries find themselves in the Donut hole each year. Often this is related to high-priced drugs like Eliquis or Xarelto, or it can be related to a variety of insulins and/or inhalers!

The Donut Hole's effect plateaued in 2020, and now what virtually happens when you're in the donut hole is that brand name medications cost you 25% of the MSRP cost until you climb out of the donut hole.

Some people will bore you with a lot of math on when you get in the donut hole and when you get out of the donut hole. I'm here to tell you, you'll drive yourself mad trying to predict it and you'll never convince your drug plan you're right and they're wrong, so this is a stress that I don't recommend my clients put on themselves!

CATASTROPHIC PHASE — In 2024, the 5% coinsurance requirement for prescription drugs in the catastrophic phase will be eliminated and Part D plans will pay 20% of total drug costs in this phase rather than 15%. In effect, this means out-of-pocket spending for Part D enrollees will be capped at $8,000. Many who enter the donut hole never actually come out on this side. If someone is on something like Revlimid for Cancer they would likely hit this pretty quickly, but otherwise they'd have to be on several midrange brand names to come out on this side and we'd probably have some other talks about drug cost savings in the interim.

PLANS OVERVIEW — Now that we have a brief understanding of what those four parts are, I want to shift gears and break down Medicare PLANS! It's important to separate the term Parts from Plans.

We just saw that we have Parts A, B, C, and D, but there is

also a Plan A, C, and D. Now I am seldom going to recommend one of those plans, but it can be confusing for someone that doesn't sit around and write legal terminology all day.

When we get into plans, we separate this into three primary types of plans: Medigap or Medicare Supplement Plans (these terms mean the same thing) A, B, C, D, F, G, K, L, M, N, and HDF/HDG (WOW, what a freaking mouth full), Medicare Advantage Plans (The same thing as Part C), Prescription drug Plans (The same thing as part D).

I hope you're following, but if not I seem to be able to loop people back in just in time so keep reading!

MEDIGAP/MEDICARE SUPPLEMENT — Let's start with these types of plans (Medicare Supplement or Medigap, remember, they're the same thing).

Remember we just said they have a whole bunch of these, but honestly we primarily use Plans F, G, and N with the rare exception of K, L, and HDF/HDG. For this book, I will focus on F, G, and N since the others are so rare they'd probably just confuse 99% of the people reading.

In 2025, a MOOP will be added to Part D.

PLAN F

The Medigap or Medicare Supplement Plan F is the most simple to explain. It fills ALL holes in Medicare Parts A and B. This includes the Part A deductible, Daily Hospital Copays, Skilled Nursing Facility Copays and it grants 365 Lifetime Reserve Hospitalization Days. It covers the Part B deductible, the 20% coinsurance, Excess Charges and also provides a Foreign Travel Emergency!

This plan is not available to anyone who became or becomes eligible for Medicare after January 1st, 2020. If you became eligible (not enrolled, but just became eligible) for Medicare before this date, you can enroll in Plan F using normal Open Enrollment, Guaranteed Issue, or Underwritten Rules as long as companies offer the plan.

PLAN G

Medigap Plan G is extremely simple once you understand what Plan F covers. Plan G is IDENTICAL to Plan F with one exception. Plan G does not cover the Part B deductible. Remember in 2024 this is the one-time $240 deductible. This deductible will go up over time, but it typically increases slowly and only once per year.

If you become eligible for Medicare after January 1st, 2020 this is most likely the Cadillac Medicare Supplement plan available to you! It also becomes your Guaranteed Issue go to plan as well. We'll cover Guaranteed Issue rules later on.

PLAN N

Medigap Plan N is used for cost savings primarily! It's also statistically the most stable on price across the board! There are however some differences in Plan N that have to be understood.

This plan also covers 100% of the hospitalization costs associated with Medicare Part A and covers the 20% coinsurance completely. It, like Plan G, does not cover the Part B deductible. The other holes are a copay for primary care and specialist appointments of UP TO $20. That's a $20 cap on the copay for each visit. There is also a $50 Emergency Room copay if you aren't admitted to the hospital. Lastly, Plan N does not cover Excess Charges. These Excess charges aren't a huge deal most of the time. Some states don't even allow them to be charged, but in states where they are charged Aetna presented a statistic that only about 4% of doctors and hospitals in the country practice charging Excess Charges.

MEDICARE ADVANTAGE
PART C

Part C of Medicare is also referred to as Medicare Advantage and the plans that you elect to fulfill this role are called Medicare Advantage PLANS, MAPDs, or MA Only Plans. These plans can get pretty complicated because there are many different types. For this book, I am going to break down the three most common plans and their pros and cons. Remember that the primary benefit to a Medicare Advantage plan is a lower cost option to having a Maximum out of Pocket on your Medicare coverage. That means you have a stop loss to stop the bleeding if you enter a catastrophic medical scenario.

PPO PLANS

This is perhaps the most common type of plan. PPO means Preferred Provider Organization. With these plans, you have reduced cost-sharing when you use a Preferred Provider or member of the PPO network. You are not however required to use a PPO provider to receive medical services.

PPO Plans typically have extra benefits like dental, vision, hearing, etc.

PPO plans normally include drug coverage.

HMO PLANS

HMO is probably the second most common Medicare Advantage Plan type. As I am saying this I am thinking nationally HMO plans could be the most common, but we most commonly used PPOs. HMO means Health Maintenance Organization. With these plans, you have an assigned Primary Care Provider and they have to refer you to doctors, hospitals, labs, and specialists within the network to receive benefits.

You may be saying, why would I limit myself to an HMO when a PPO is available.

Well, here's why. If you normally use a pretty tight group of doctors and hospitals anyway, they're in the HMO network, and you don't travel a ton, you can get an HMO and you typically have much lower copays, deductibles, coinsurance, and other cost-sharing parameters as well as the ever-coveted EXTRA BENEFITS like Dental, Vision, Hearing, Rides to Doctors, Chiropractic Visits, and Over the Counter Benefits.

Yes, PPO plans often offer some of these benefits as well, but HMOs expand the benefits with money that would normally be used for larger networks.

HMOs also normally include drug coverage with them.

MSA PLANS

I wanted to add MSA plans because they are often extremely valuable for certain types of people. This type of person is normally very healthy, financially stable (not rich necessarily), and has a positive outlook on the future.

MSA stands for Medicare Savings Account. These plans are high deductible health plans with an annual deposit that can build up an account value that will eventually eclipse the deductible and provide someone with 100% coverage. They have the added benefit of normally being a $0 premium, accepted at all providers that accept Traditional Medicare, and the growing account value can be used for any IRS qualified healthcare expense including, dental, vision, hearing, etc.

The cons of these would be that if you have health problems that arise too quickly you can spend more than is on the account and the deductible would cause you to have a substantial out-of-pocket amount. Another con is you still have to buy a stand-alone part D plan, but your MSA Account Value can be used towards Drug Copays!

HOSPITAL INDEMNITY PLANS

Sometimes we recommend a Hospital Indemnity Plan with riders that are designed to fill the holes in Medicare Advantage Plans! These plans are often extremely valuable!

One of the things we commonly recommend is an MSA plan with a Hospital Indemnity Plan with a lump sum cancer rider until the account value on the MSA plan has reached a level that wouldn't require you to have that HIP plan in place anymore and then you can shed it! This is like a vanishing premium!

SEPARATE PLANS

Dental, Vision and Hearing

When someone chooses a Medigap Plan, they normally don't have non-medical Dental, Vision, and Hearing coverage. When they ask about these benefits we recommend a couple of different plans depending on their needs. Mostly Nationwide and Manhattan Life fulfill these needs the best.

Most of the time these plans have one-year waiting periods on major services, so we consider the long-term solutions. We don't sell them as a quick fix to a big problem. They're a long-term fix to your dental, vision, and hearing needs.

Another thing with these benefits to consider is that with Medicare Advantage you often have some of these included but it may not be a bad idea to have one of these plans to give you a boost in coverage!

ADDITIONAL CANCER COVERAGE

We always recommend a lump sum cancer plan for our clients. Here are the 2 situations it's needed.

One, if you have Medicare Advantage plans, you typically have to pay 20% of your outpatient Chemotherapy or Radiation until you have met your maximum out of pocket (which is normally around $4000-10,000). So, a $10,000 lump sum cancer can cover that for one calendar year for you.

Two, Medicare's drug coverage can leave major holes for a lot of high-priced cancer medication, which is more and more often being used instead of outpatient radiation. These medications can cost someone $10,000 - $15,000 a year.

At a minimum, we recommend a $10,000 lump sum cancer policy for our clients, but a bigger one, up to say $50,000, would not be a bad idea at all!

PART 2

ENROLLMENT PERIODS

OPEN ENROLLMENT

Now, here is a term that often gets used for periods that it doesn't apply to!

Open Enrollment can mean a couple of different things, but with Medicare, it has two distinct periods that apply.

One, the Medigap Open Enrollment period. This is the period of time that is 6 months before and 6 months after your 65th birthday and/or your. Part B effective date. It gives you the right to purchase a Medigap policy with no health questions.

OPEN ENROLLMENT PERIOD

(OEP)

Also, January 1st to March 31st is the OEP or Open Enrollment Period. This one is different. This is for people to make one of the following elections:

Medicare Advantage back to Traditional Medicare

Medicare Advantage to another "like" Medicare Advantage plan.

This period is for untangling bad decisions made during AEP (Annual Election Period).

ANNUAL ELECTION PERIOD

(AEP)

This is the big period that gets advertised on TV and everywhere honestly! This period is October 15th to December 7th, but October 1st through 14th is called Pre-AEP.

Pre-AEP is when new year plan information can be presented but not sold. AEP is when it can be sold or enrolled in for the following calendar year.

All elections during this period warrant a January 1st effective date.

Things that this election period can do:

- PDP or Part D plan swaps
- Medicare to Medicare Advantage
- Medicare Advantage Disenrollment
- Medicare Advantage to Medicare Advantage plans
- Medicare Supplements can be shopped during this period, but no special rules apply. They must still be underwritten

UNDERWRITING

Medigap plans require underwriting (answering health questions) to change from one plan to another to get a better price or different Plan. This is of course when someone is outside of their Medicare Supplement Open Enrollment Period that is 6 months from the 65th birthday or Part B effective date.

Hospital indemnity and Cancer insurance can use underwriting criteria as well.

The underwriting criteria can be vastly different from company to company on all of these products.

As an example, Mutual of Omaha only goes back 2 years on cancer treatment in their look back but Aetna goes back 3. However, Aetna will consider someone with mild COPD and Mutual of Omaha will instantly decline their application.

There is one exception to this, guaranteed issue periods.

GUARANTEED ISSUE

(GI)

GI Periods as they pertain to Medicare are mostly related to Medicare Supplements.

Here are some Medigap or Medicare Supplement Guaranteed Issue examples:

1. Someone who isn't in Open Enrollment because they're over 65 and outside of 6 months from their Part B effective date who has maintained other credible coverage and is no voluntarily or involuntarily (depending on the state's laws on this) losing that credible coverage (most commonly through retirement). They would have a 63 day Guaranteed Issue period starting the day that they lost that coverage to get a Medigap plan without answering health questions. Also, remember as we discussed before, they can only get certain types of Medigap plans - Plan F is commonly used in this situation for people who were initially eligible for Medicare before January 1st, 2020 and Plan G for people who were eligible after January 1st, 2020.

2. Someone who is on a Medicare Advantage plan but moved out of the plan's area of availability would typically be given a guaranteed issue period which could also be used to purchase a Medigap plan.

3. Certain states have an Anniversary Rule or Birthday Rule guaranteed issue laws where they can change every year without answering health questions.

SPECIAL ENROLLMENT PERIOD

(SEP)

Similar to Guaranteed Issue rules, there are certain times you can use what's called a SEP to enroll in drug plans or Medicare Advantage Plans due to some of the reasons we discussed in the Guaranteed Issue chapter.

INITIAL ENROLLMENT PERIOD

(IEP)

I tend to do things backward. If you have made it to the IEP chapter you're reaching the end, but most people start with this one.

The IEP is the period when you're turning 65 or first becoming Medicare Eligible that starts 3 months before the first month of eligibility, encompasses the first month of eligibility, and ends 3 months after that month. It's a 7 month period!

During this period you can pretty much do anything. It normally overlaps your Medigap Open Enrollment Period so you can get Medigap plans, Medicare Advantage Plans, Part D Prescription Plans, etc.

This is a good time to get set up the right way so you don't have to use as many of the other periods we discussed.

H_2O

When a child looks at the chemical compound of water, they probably think it's just a typo or misprint, but when an adult looks at it they instantly think water.

When I look at (A+B)+G+D) I think Medicare beneficiaries set up RIGHT. But I can also see (A+B)+N+D) and think that! By the same accord, I can think this way about (A+B)<C+HIP given the right circumstances.

Whereas there is only one way to make water, there are multiple ways to satisfy someone's Medicare needs, and it honestly all depends on their circumstances.

Now that we have broken down Medicare in general, I will share with you a co-authored informational piece called "How to Avoid 7 Costly Mistakes with Medicare".

Part 3

HOW TO *AVOID* 7 COSTLY MISTAKES WITH MEDICARE

MISTAKE #1

MISSING ENROLLMENT DEADLINES

Failing to timely enroll in your Medicare plan is a costly error that can result in life-long penalties and/or denial of your application for coverage. Enrolling in Medicare Part B too early can cost you thousands of dollars in premiums for coverage you cannot use, so here is what you need to know.

INITIAL ENROLLMENT AT 65

If you are drawing social security benefits at least 4 months before you turn 65, your enrollment for Part A (Hospital) and Part B (Medical) should happen automatically, and you should receive your card before your birthday month. If you are not receiving social security benefits when you turn 65 and are not covered under a large group health plan, you must take action to enroll. You can visit your local Social Security office or save time by enrolling online at www.ssa. gov/benefits/medicare.

There is a seven-month Initial Enrollment Period when you turn 65. This enrollment window begins three months before your birthday month and ends 3 months after.

Enrollment in Medicare consists of three different insurance plans or Medicare Advantage:

- Part A – Covers inpatient hospital care, skilled nursing (not to be confused with nursing home care), hospice care, and some home health care.

- Part B – Covers outpatient care, medical supplies, doctors and surgeons, and preventative care. (Sometimes covers prescription medications like those administered through pumps.)

- Part C – Covers Medicare Parts A, B, and sometimes Part D in one plan – also called Medicare Advantage (not the same as a Medigap policy)

Failure to sign up within the enrollment period can result in a penalty (10% per year for Part B and 12% per year on Part D) being added to your premium for each year you were not enrolled after becoming eligible.

Example: Fred turns 65 in July, is no longer working, and has not yet drawn any social security benefits. Fred wants to be proactive and enrolls in Medicare. He has a seven-month enrollment window from April 1st through October 31st. Fred contacts Bobby Brock Insurance in May so his coverage can begin the first day of the month he turns 65. A qualified Medicare specialist assists Fred in signing up for Medicare and enrolling in a Medicare Part D drug plan and a Medigap insurance policy. Fred also elects to purchase a cancer insurance policy and a dental vision & hearing plan.

ANNUAL ELECTION PERIOD & MEDICARE ADVANTAGE

OPEN ENROLLMENT PERIOD

Each year, there is an Annual Election Period, which runs from October 15th through December 7th. During this time, Medicare beneficiaries have the opportunity to make changes to their Medicare coverage. They may switch from Original Medicare to Medicare Advantage, or from Medicare Advantage to Original Medicare. They may also change their Medicare Part D plan. There is no limit on how many times they can make changes during this period.

If after selecting a new Medicare Advantage Plan during the Annual Enrollment Period you are unhappy with it, all is not lost. You will have another opportunity to switch your plan during the Medicare Advantage Open Enrollment Period (MA OEP). MA OEP runs from January 1st through March 31st. Under the new rule established in 2018, the MA OEP was extended to March 31st... The new rule also allows you to switch to another MA plan. Any changes will go into effect on the first day of the next month after you enroll. The MA OEP is the time when you can change to another Medicare Advantage Plan or Original Medicare with or without a Part D Prescription plan.

Medigap insurance does not have to be changed during the Annual Election Period. You can apply to change Medigap plans at any time; however, you must be medically underwritten unless you are in the Initial Open Enrollment Period or qualified for a Special Enrollment Period, which will be discussed further in a moment.

LATE ENROLLMENT

If Fred had missed his Initial Enrollment Period of the seven-month window mentioned before, he must wait until the General Enrollment Period for Part B (Medical) and the Annual Election Period for Part D.

For Medicare Part B (Medical), Fred's enrollment would be delayed until the next General Enrollment period. The General Enrollment period runs January 1st through March 31st each year, and the coverage would begin on the following July 1st. His Part B premium would have a penalty for life equal to 10% of the Part B premium for each year he went without the coverage but was entitled to it.

For Medicare Part D (prescriptions), Fred's enrollment is delayed until the next Annual Election period which runs from October 15th through December 7th for a January 1st effective date. Fred's premium would be penalized 1% for every month he was entitled to the coverage, but did not have it. The penalty is permanent.

Late enrollment in Part A (Hospital) can be done anytime after you turn 65, and there is no penalty for those who get it free. Medicare Part A does not have a premium if the beneficiary or their spouse paid Medicare employment taxes during the years leading up to Medicare. People who are required to pay a premium for Part A will have a 10% penalty. The penalty is not permanent. It would last for twice the number of years the beneficiary was eligible for Part A but did not have it.

SPECIAL ENROLLMENT PERIODS

Special Enrollment Periods allow beneficiaries to enroll without a penalty. The following are some common examples that qualify you for special enrollment:

Example: Fred was covered under a large group plan,

which was his primary coverage. He leaves his job and loses his coverage effective January 1.

- He has 8 months to sign up on Medicare Parts A & B,
- 2 months to sign up on Part D, and
- 63 days to apply for Medigap policy without answering health questions.

Note: If Fred delayed enrollment in his Medicare Part B because he had primary coverage through a group plan, he preserved his 6 months open enrollment period for Medigap. This gives him 6 months instead of 63 days to enroll in a Medigap plan without answering any health questions.

Fred was covered by a Medicare Advantage Plan or a Part D prescription plan and moved out of the plan's service area. (Fred has two months to enroll in another Medicare Advantage Plan, Part D plan, or return to Original Medicare and enroll in a Medigap policy without having to answer health questions. The two months begin the date of the move or the date he notifies his plan of the move, if later.)

Fred qualifies for Extra Help for Medicare Prescription coverage or has Medicaid. He can switch his Medicare prescription drug plan or Medicare Advantage Plan one time each calendar quarter but is not entitled to enroll in a Medigap policy without answering health questions.

MISTAKE #2

MISSING THE MEDIGAP OPEN ENROLLMENT PERIOD

Medicare supplements, also called Medigap insurance, are designed to pay some of the deductibles, co-pays, and the 20% coinsurance that Medicare Parts A & B do not cover. There are 11 distinct plans, plus select plans, but the most currently popular are designated the letters F, G & N.

Many insurance companies sell these plans, but there can be no difference in benefits from company to company. This is due to a 1992 rule passed by the National Association of Insurance Commissioners' which standardized Medigap policies to make them easier to compare. Although the benefits of plan G, for example, must be identical across all companies, there can be, and often are, vast differences in monthly premiums and service.

To qualify for a Medigap plan, there is a one-time, six-month "Open Enrollment" that occurs when you enroll in Medicare Part B or turn 65. This Open Enrollment is the only time you are allowed to enroll in a Medigap policy without answering health questions unless you qualify for a Special Enrollment Period. Once the Open Enrollment window has expired, you can be turned down for coverage, or you may have to buy a more expensive policy from a company that will accept a person with particular medical problems.

You are allowed to enroll in a Medigap policy up to six months ahead of your Part B effective date, but the coverage would begin the month your Medicare Part B begins. Alternatively, you may enroll up to five months after the month you turn 65 for the coverage to begin on the first day of the following month. You may apply for any Medigap policy you want anytime during this period without answering any health questions, and you cannot be denied coverage.

Example: Fred turns 65 July 5th and enrolls in Medicare Parts A & B with a July 1st effective date, but he forgets to enroll in a Medigap policy. Fred had a window of 6 months before July 1st and 5 months after July. He applies for a Medigap plan in January of the following year. Fred has to answer "yes" to the health question about heart or circulatory surgery, so he is turned down for most plans. One plan will take Fred, but the premium is 100% higher than it would have been had he applied during open enrollment. Fred made a big mistake by missing the Open Enrollment Deadline for Medigap.

MISTAKE #3

ENROLLING IN MEDICARE PART B TOO EARLY

Medicare Part B is primary medical coverage. If you are working past 65 and your group insurance plan has over 20 employees, you may not need Medicare Part B, because your group policy would be your primary coverage. If you enroll in Part B unnecessarily, you are paying a premium every month for insurance you do not need and you are wasting money on a premium for insurance you cannot use. What's more, by enrolling in Part B when you didn't need it you have used your six-month open enrollment period unnecessarily.

> Example: Fred went to the social security office when he turned 65 on July 5th, 2015. Fred was ill-advised to enroll in Medicare Parts A and B. He should not have enrolled in Part B, because he was still working and had primary coverage through his employer's group plan. Three years later Fred retired due to an illness. Fred is eligible for a 63 day guaranteed issue period to enroll in Medigap without answering health questions, but not the 6 months open enrollment period because the Open Enrollment began when he enrolled in Part B. Not only did he waste his 6 months Open Enrollment Period, but Fred also wasted over $4000 paying Part B premiums for coverage

he couldn't use. If Fred applies within 63 days of losing his coverage he is guaranteed eligibility for a Medigap Plan F. Others with Medicare eligibility after January 1, 2020, would be guaranteed Medigap Plan G.

MISTAKE #4

FAILING TO APPLY FOR THE LOW INCOME SUBSIDY

Medicare provides a program for people with limited income and resources to help cover their prescription drug costs. "Extra Help" bridges this gap for those who qualify, and it can greatly reduce the financial burden of those who need financial assistance. Some people qualify for Extra Help automatically, and others will have to apply. Your eligibility for extra help is based on your income and your state's individual requirements.

For example, in 2023 in the state of Mississippi, if you are single, your monthly income must be less than $1,508 to receive this subsidy. For a married couple, the monthly income amount must be less than $2,022.

This subsidy is an often overlooked benefit that can reduce your Part D premiums, waive your Part D deductibles, and also lower your Part D co-pays.

MISTAKE #5

MISTAKING MEDICARE ADVANTAGE FOR MEDIGAP

One of the most common mistakes people make is confusing Medicare Advantage plans with Medigap policies. It is important you understand the distinction between Medicare Advantage and Medigap policies because the benefits are vastly different. Typically, the price for an Advantage plan is cheaper than that of a Medigap policy, but your out-of-pocket responsibility is greater. In some geographical areas and for some people, Medicare Advantage plans work great. But they are not appropriate for everyone.

REMEMBER THIS RULE OF THUMB:

Don't buy a plan for the Premium, buy it for the overall value which includes benefits, premiums, and provider network!

Understand what you are buying! Most of our clients who live in rural areas prefer to buy a Medigap policy if they are medically qualified. These plans are more widely accepted by doctors and they leave very little for the insured to pay out of their own pockets.

In some areas, Medicare Advantage plans are a more attractive option. These areas commonly include urban areas where there are competing healthcare systems.

In the event that someone cannot afford or does not qualify for a Medigap policy, an Advantage plan may be the most attractive option. For these folks, Medicare Advantage Plan might be a good alternative, because co-pays are more affordable than Original Medicare alone. Also, Advantage Plans do provide an out-of-pocket limit each year. The out-of-pocket limit can be quite high – up to $10,000 per year unless you qualify for Medicaid. You should always consider the plan's network because some doctors may not accept these plans.

MEDICARE ADVANTAGE PLANS contain all the basic benefits of Medicare Parts A, B, & sometimes D. There are several types of Advantage plans, but the two most common to be discussed are HMOs and PPOs.

HMOs are Health Maintenance Organizations that pay fees to particular medical providers to treat plan members. Members are required to pay co-pays and some coinsurance until they reach the annual individual out-of-pocket limit.

HMOs are generally more competitive in large metropolitan areas where several hospital systems can compete for patients. The doctors and hospitals in the plan have to agree to provide member services for a lower cost and in return, the plan refers patients to the providers.

HMO members are assigned a primary care doctor who must be seen before being referred to specialists. The primary care doctor is responsible for overseeing the care of the patient. HMO members must see plan doctors to receive benefits, except in emergency cases. This can be a big disadvantage if your provider is not in the HMO.

PPOs are Preferred Provider Organizations. These are Medicare Advantage Plans with a network of providers who have agreed to discount services for the plan, but the plan still provides benefits if you go outside the network. However, going outside this network may require additional costs and exposes you to higher out-of-pocket limits.

The premiums of HMO and PPO plans can be very low, and in some cases the premium can be $0, making them very attractive from that standpoint. If you opt for Medicare Advantage, you must be comfortable with the potential out-of-pocket costs and restrictive networks.

MISTAKE #6

FAILURE TO INSURE WHAT'S NOT COVERED BY MEDICARE

Do not assume that Medicare covers everything. In fact, there are several areas commonly overlooked that warrant important consideration. Here are a few areas that may not be sufficiently covered by Medicare:

CANCER TREATMENT — Medicare's website warns consumers that doctors may recommend services not covered by Medicare for which they would be solely responsible. Some cancer treatment drugs are extremely expensive and may not be covered or may only partially be covered. You should consider buying a lump sum cancer insurance policy in addition to your Medicare coverage.

LONG TERM CARE — Medicare covers some short-term skilled nursing care limited to recovery services. This does not cover long-term custodial care, such as nursing homes or assisted living. Consider Long Term Care Insurance in addition to your Medicare coverage.

DEDUCTIBLES, COPAYS, AND COINSURANCE — Medicare alone still requires you to pay deductibles, copays, and coinsurance for which you are responsible. For 2024 they are:

- Part A (Hospital) deductible is $1,632 per 60 day benefit period.
- Part A (Hospital) daily hospital copay beginning on day 61 is $408 and up to $816 per day on the 91st day. No coverage remains after day 150.
- Skilled Nursing facility copays of $204 per day for days 21-100. No coverage after 100 days.
- Part B (Medical) deductible of $240 per calendar year (2024).
- 20% coinsurance on Part B medical expenses with no limit to your out-of-pocket expenses.

MEDIGAP INSURANCE POLICIES pay most of these Medicare-approved costs not covered by Medicare. Plan F pays all these listed costs in #3, whereas Plan G pays all but the $240 Part B deductible.

MEDIGAP SELECT PLANS are like standard plans, except you must use a network hospital to keep from paying the $1,632 Inpatient Deductible. Rural areas do not usually have network hospitals. The premiums on select plans are a little lower, but not worth the requirement of using a specific hospital to have your deductible paid.

MEDICARE ADVANTAGE PLANS have different benefit structures and provide an annual out-of-pocket limit of up to $11,500, however, most plans do not have out-of-pocket limits that high. There is no insurance designed to pay the copays on Medicare Advantage Plans, and Advantage Plans are not Medicare supplemental insurance policies. Medigap policies cannot be used with Medicare Advantage plans, however, there are other supplemental health policies that can help offset some out-of-pocket costs. Cancer, heart attack, stroke, and hospital indemnity policies are available if you qualify.

MISTAKE #7

NOT ANNUALLY REVIEWING YOUR MEDICARE DRUG PLAN

Not reviewing your Part D coverage on a yearly basis is a big mistake that is also very frequently made. Many people assume that since their Medicare Part D prescription coverage has been good, there is no need to review or change it. Some people keep their existing Drug Plan through the Annual Election Period only to find out in January the premiums and copays have increased. Furthermore, the plan can revise covered drugs, copays, and can add new restrictions such as step therapy or quantity limits on prescriptions. Changes would have to wait until the next Annual Election Period.

Our Medicare advisors use special tools to help you review, compare benefits, and choose your plan each year. We take care of the enrollment for you and assist you if there is an issue with your enrollment. Don't wait until the last minute! Our clients are reminded to review annually via our websites and mail.

The best way to proceed if you're already on a Medicare plan but aren't sure you have what's best for you because of price or maybe coverage, or if you're someone who is turning 65, retiring, or becoming eligible for disability

Medicare, is to reach out to me through any of my mediums!

CONCLUSION

I train thousands of agents how to do this, but I am consistently helping people make their individual choices as well. I think we need more qualified and helpful Medicare-focused insurance agents. Not cold calling plan flippers that aren't there to help, but true problem solvers that can take your circumstance and come up with a simple and appropriate solution.

ABOUT THE AUTHOR

Justin Brock is one of the foremost resources on all things Medicare and Health Insurance. He owns and operates multiple companies that serve both Medicare and Health Insurance consumers and agents focused on serving those markets. Bobby Brock Insurance is a National Medicare and Health Insurance agency that has served over 50,000 Medicare and Health Insurance beneficiaries.

With thousands of five star reviews and an award winning team, Justin's team at Bobby Brock Insurance can be trusted to help with any problem that arises. In a world where there are a ton of low value proposition Medicare and Health Insurance focused agents and organizations, Justin's team is a breath of fresh air.

Made in United States
Orlando, FL
20 September 2024

51709268R00030